4.95

Echinacea:
The Immune Herb!

D1431116

Recycle
Conserve

This book is printed on Simpson 60lb recycled paper .

Botanica Press, Capitola, CA

**Other books in the "Herbs and Health" series
by Christopher Hobbs:**

Milk Thistle–The Liver Herb

Medicinal Mushrooms

Usnea: The Herbal Antibiotic

Natural Liver Therapy

Vitex: The Female Herb

Ginkgo: Elixir of Youth

Foundations of Health

5th Printing February 1994

Copyright September, 1990
by Christopher Hobbs

Michael Miovic and
Beth Baugh, copy editors
Illustrations: Christopher Hobbs (figs. 1B, 3, 5, 6, 7)
                Cover Photo by Richard Hamilton Smith
                Mark Johnson (fig. 4)
                Steven Foster (fig. 1A)

Botanica Press
Box 742
Capitola, CA 95010

TABLE OF CONTENTS

ECHINACEA
THE IMMUNE HERB!

SUMMARY

This booklet presents up-to-date practical information on the use of *echinacea*—an important herb for infections, colds, flu, and a host of other major and minor ailments. Specific instructions are included for the following:

- ✔ Which ailments echinacea works for
- ✔ Choosing the best echinacea products
- ✔ How much to take and for how long
- ✔ Children's dosages

All of this will be backed up with solid scientific evidence, for echinacea is the place where past and present meet, where traditional wisdom and modern research fully agree.

INTRODUCTION

In the 1870's, a doctor in Pawnee City, Nebraska made an unusual challenge to a couple of Eastern doctors. Convinced of the healing power of *echinacea*, an herb he had learned of from local Indians, he offered to let himself be bitten by a rattlesnake and to cure himself with nothing but this plant. The doctors declined his challenge and lived to regret it. Within a generation, echinacea (pronounced *eke-<u>nay</u>-shuh*) had become the most

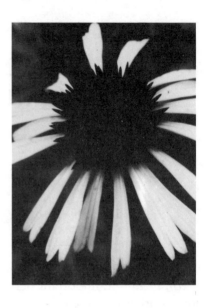

(A) *Echinacea angustifolia*

Shorter ray petals that do not droop. The roots of this species are commonly used. Native to the plains states.

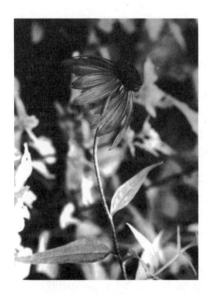

(B) *Echinacea purpurea*

Longer, dark purple ray petals. The tops and roots are used. Native to the eastern U.S. Easy to cultivate in a variety of climates.

Fig. 1   The two main commercial species of echinacea

The most widely encountered common name for echinacea is **Purple Coneflower**, for obvious reasons—the plant is bright purple and has a large, cone-shaped projection in the middle of the flower.

Other common names:

Purple Kansas Coneflower,

Black Sampson,

Red Sunflower,

Comb Flower,

Cock Up Hat,

Missouri Snakeroot,

Indian Head and

Kansas Snakeroot.[1]

prescribed herbal medicine in the United States, not only for poisoning, but for a wide range of infectious diseases.

Doctors initially marvelled that a single herb could affect so many different conditions—and without side effects. But echinacea's amazing action was eventually explained with the discovery of the immune system, because the herb strengthens the body's ability to

---

The national average is 2.4 colds per year per person—or over 600 million cases in all.

---

resist infection and poisoning. This has been scientifically confirmed time and again. Since 1930, over 300 journal articles have appeared verifying the effectiveness of echinacea. Today the herb is sold widely throughout Europe and the United States, both in prescription and over-the-counter forms.

Millions of people get colds and flu every year in the United States. The national average is 2.4 colds per year per person—or over 600 million cases in all. Add to this all the other common stresses of modern living—car exhaust, pollution, pesticides, deforestation,

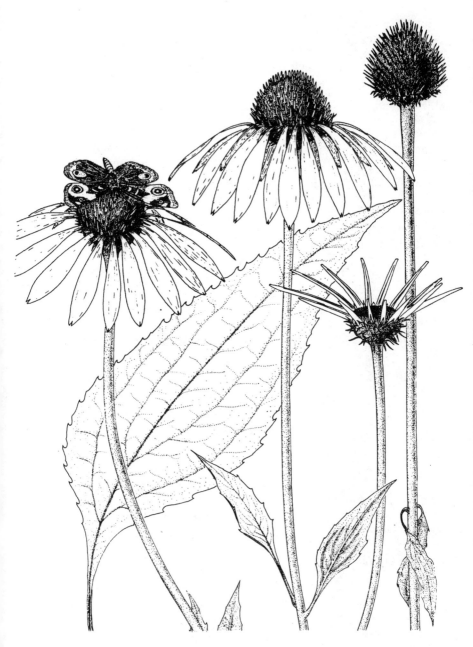

Fig. 2   Echinacea purpurea

chemical wastes from industry, drug-abuse, crime, and plain old fast-living—and you can see why now, more than ever, we need to take good care of our immune systems. There are so many things in our environment today that disrupt the body's age-old processes. Nor can we just down antibiotics forever, because when our immune systems are not working well, antibiotics can only postpone the inevitable.

So if you are intrigued by the possibility of fewer colds and flu, and want to learn about an effective natural alternative to antibiotics for treating skin, gum, and urinary tract infections—to name just a few—then read on! Ten years ago few herbalists in this country had little idea how to use echinacea or even what it was. However, some far-sighted herbalists began importing echinacea products and manufacturing liquid extracts from wildcrafted American herb. Today it is one of the most popular herbs ever, and it is growing more popular as the cold seasons tick by.

THE HISTORY OF ECHINACEA

Echinacea is native to the plains of the United States. It grows wild nowhere else in the world, except for a few sparse patches in southern Canada. So naturally the first people to use this herb were the Native American Indians. Samples of echinacea have been found in archaeological digs of American Indian sites dating back to the 1600's.

The Native American Indians were often skilled herbalists. Of the hundreds of herbs commonly used by the various Indian nations during the 17th and 18th centuries, several stand out. They used ginseng for digestion, golden seal for wounds and infections, sassafras as a spring tonic, slippery elm for soothing the respiratory and digestive tracts, and senega snakeroot for bronchial congestion. These herbs all played an important role in pioneer medicine, and the first four are still in high demand today.

But the Plains Indians revered echinacea above all other herbs and found many uses for it (see Table 1).[2,3] For alleviating toothaches, sore throats, coughs, infections, snakebites and numerous other diseases and afflictions, there was no better medicine. Interestingly, one of the Indians' preferred methods of

Table 1

AMERICAN INDIAN USES OF ECHINACEA

TRIBE	AREA	USES
CHEYENNE	Colorado, Kansas	sore mouth, gums, etc.
CHOCTAWS	Mississippi, Alabama	coughs, dyspepsia
COMANCHE	northern Texas	toothache, sore throat
CROW	Montana, Wyoming	colds, toothache, colic
DAKOTA (Oglala)	South Dakota	inflammations
DELAWARE	southern New York	gonorrhea
HIDATSA	—	stimulates energy
KIOWA	southwestern Kansas	coughs, sore throat
MESKWAKI (Fox)	southern Wisconsin	cramps, fits
OMAHA	eastern Nebraska	septic diseases, etc.
OMAHA-PONCA	northern Nebraska	as an eye-wash
PAWNEE	central Nebraska	children's game
SIOUX (Dakota)	northern Nebraska South Dakota	bowels, tonsillitis hydrophobia, sepsis
WINNEBAGO	eastern Wisconsin	anesthetic against heat

taking echinacea was to suck on a piece of the root all day. The effectiveness of this practice seems to be corroborated by German researchers who feel that echinacea liquid extracts may begin stimulating immune tissue in the mouth as soon as they are taken.(see fig. 4, p.18)[4]

The Purple Coneflower was known to European botanists as early as the 1690's, and the botanist Moench named the genus *Echinacea* in 1794, from the Greek echinos (sea urchin or hedgehog), referring to the plant's sea urchin-like cone. However, the Europeans knew nothing about echinacea's medicinal properties—or about the properties of any other New World plants for that matter. They had to learn everything from the American Indians, who were quite friendly and willing to share their considerable knowledge with the first pioneers. Books and articles from the early 18th century show that although the settlers brought with them a few herbs (such as plantain), for the most part they had little knowledge of medicinal plants and a great need for them.

"...he offered to come to Cincinnati and.... allow a rattlesnake of our selection to bite him wherever we might prefer.... proposing then to antidote the poison by means of Echinacea only."

But echinacea did not really become renowned until the advent of H.C.F. Meyer, the German lay physician of Pawnee City, Nebraska, mentioned in the introduction. It was Meyer who, around 1870, formulated and began selling a patent medicine containing echinacea (and other herbs such as hops and wormwood) that became quite popular. Meyer unmodestly named his formula "Meyer's Blood Purifier." After sixteen years of experimenting with his preparation, he became thoroughly convinced of its efficacy. He wrote to two eminent medical men of the time, Dr. John King and John Uri Lloyd, and made his now-famous claim that echinacea could cure snakebites.

King and Lloyd belonged to the "Eclectic" school of medicine; that is, they favored the use of herbs in clinical practice. The Eclectic doctors were quite active and influential in the United States from the mid 1800's up through the 1930's. Lloyd later described Meyer's overture as follows:

"In view of our incredulity as to the virtues of the drug in the direction of the bites of poisonous serpents, he offered to come to Cincinnati and, in the presence of a committee selected by ourselves, allow a rattlesnake of our selection to bite him wherever we might prefer the wound to be inflicted, proposing then to antidote the poison by means of Echinacea only. This offer (or rather, challenge) we declined. Dr. Meyer, thinking this was because we had no serpent at our command, again offered not only to come to Cincinnati and submit to the ordeal formerly proposed, but to bring with him a full-sized rattlesnake, possessed of its natural fangs..."[5]

King and Lloyd also dismissed this second offer as quackery, much to their regret. Echinacea was introduced into the materia medica by 1887 and only twenty years later had become the most popular herb among both the Eclectic and regular medical doctors. In fact, it was King and Lloyd who eventually championed the cause of echinacea. Although the herb was always surrounded with controversy, and the American Medical Association never officially accepted it, still many doctors used echinacea faithfully.

The Eclectics used echinacea for many complaints. They employed it as a digestive stimulant and also considered it to be an excellent blood purifier. The plant's immune stimulating properties were first noticed by Unruh around 1914. By then the Eclectics knew that echinacea increased the activity of the *phagocytes*—immune cells that must disarm and recycle bacteria and waste materials in the body. Dr. A. L. Nourse published the following comment in the American Journal of Clinical Medicine in 1914:

"So far as my own experience is concerned, I will state that for conditions requiring strengthening of the reparative forces of the body—raising the opsonic index—I know of no agent of greater value than Echinacea....good for anything requiring the police-powers of the individual to be increased."

The "opsonic index" measures the level of antibodies present in the blood that can render bacteria and other cells susceptible to phagocytosis (engulfment). To be more precise, one could say

Echinacea: History at a Glance

- Pre-1800's
Echinacea is an important medicine for many Native American Indian tribes.
- 1690's
European botanists first classify echinacea.
- 1870
Meyer learns of echinacea from Indians in Pawnee City, Nebraska and makes "Meyer's Blood Purifier."
- 1887
Meyer offers to let himself be bitten by a rattlesnake in order to prove echinacea's curative powers.
- 1891
The first article on echinacea appears in a medical journal.
- 1902
Echinacea is adopted for use by homeopathic doctors. 200,000 pounds of echinacea are marketed in the U.S.
- 1907
Echinacea is the most popular herb in medical practice in

(continued on next page)

that the term "blood purifier" signifies a medicine that increases the body's powers of elimination and stimulates immune functions such as phagocytosis.

Dr. Finley Ellingwood, a popular Eclectic doctor and author of the time, had this to say about echinacea:

> "For from twenty to twenty-five years, Echinacea has been passing through the stages of critical experimentation under the observation of several thousand physicians, and its remarkable properties are receiving positive confirmation. As yet, but few disparaging statements have been made. All who use it correctly fall quickly into line as enthusiasts in its praise; the experience of the writer is similar to that of the rest."

Ellingwood recommended echinacea especially for boils, abscesses, pain of breast cancer, poison oak, insect and scorpion bites, tetanus, colds, and urinary tract infections.[6]

Around 1902, echinacea began to gain recognition among the Homeopaths, a school of doctors that believed the axiom that "like cures like." Homeopathic medicines are often given in moderate to high dilution. Under the influence of the Homeopaths, echinacea quickly became popular for general weakness, wounds that would not heal, and as a stimulant for the whole body. It may have been the Homeopaths who introduced echinacea into European medicine, where it has been highly regarded ever since. In the 1930's, German preparations of echinacea became popular, and several of them are still manufactured today.

As the interest in Echinacea has increased, hundreds of scientific studies have been conducted, and numerous medicinal products containing the herb have been made available to the public. Since the early 1930's, the United States has exported over 50,000 pounds of echinacea annually to European markets, and beginning in the late 1970's, herbal manufacturers began making domestic products. Today, nearly every herbal company has one or more echinacea products—it has developed into one of the top-selling herbs of all time.

MODERN VERIFICATION OF TRADITIONAL USES

Pharmacology

In scientific terms, one of the most interesting aspects of herbology is pharmacology—the study of how a given medicinal substance affects the body on a biochemical level. This kind of

the U.S., among both Eclectic and regular medical doctors.
• 1910
Echinacea is recognized as an immune stimulant that increases the attack of white blood cells on bacteria and waste material.
• 1930
Echinacea preparations become popular in Germany.
1930's-1980's
More than 400 scientific journal articles appear exploring the medicinal properties of echinacea. About 50,000 pounds of echinacea are exported annually from the U.S. to European markets.
• 1980
U.S. herbalists "rediscover" echinacea.
• 1986
More than 240 medicinal products in Germany have echinacea as a constituent. In the U.S., echinacea consumption quadruples over previous year and more than 100,000 pounds of the herb are sold.[7]

investigation attracts considerable funding from various commercial enterprises which want to develop and market new medicinal products. Consequently extensive research has been conducted on echinacea. The general conclusion is that it boosts the immune system by increasing the body's ability to ward off, fight, and dispose of bacterial and viral infections. Table 2 summarizes the major physiological effects of echinacea. The information is drawn from over 300 published research papers.

One of the most prevalent uses of echinacea is to forestall or shorten the common cold, flu, and related ailments. Surprisingly, though, few studies have been conducted on this subject, despite the fact that so much research has been done on other aspects of echinacea's activity. It is encouraging that the few studies carried out have given positive results. For instance, in one experiment, 109 children aged 3-5 received a preparation containing echinacea (and 2 other herbs), while 100 did not. The children who received the preparation with echinacea had fewer days of fever and sickness than the control group.[8]

Subsequent controlled studies on children confirmed and amplified these initial results. The same preparation with echinacea proved to be a protective and curative agent for infections of the upper respiratory tract,[9] as well as for viral infections.[10] A similar preparation which contained echinacea and boneset herb demonstrated success in fighting influenza and upper respiratory infections.[11] Of course, it would be more conclusive if the studies were done with echinacea alone, but they can be considered an important step in the study of Echinacea.

Major Active Constituents

The observation of *what* a plant does to the body is one thing, but figuring out exactly *how* it does it can be much more complex. The mechanisms by which pure drug substances cause certain effects are difficult enough to study, sometimes requiring years to pinpoint. Imagine then trying to study an herbal substance, which contains a whole array of different chemical compounds that work together to bring about delicate changes within the body! What researchers have to do is patiently isolate

Table 2

Echinacea's Major Physiological Effects

- **Stimulates the leukocytes** (white blood cells that help fight infection).

- **Increases "phagocytic power" of the immune cells** (enhances the body's ability to dispose of bacteria, infected and damaged cells, and harmful chemicals).

- **Hyaluronidase inhibition** (this helps protect cells during infection, and prevents pathogens, bacteria, and viruses from entering in the first place).

- **Mild antibiotic effect**

- **Stimulates the growth of healthy, new tissue**

- **Antiphlogistic/anti-inflammatory effect** (helps to reduce soreness, redness, and other symptoms of infection).

- **Stimulates the properdin/complement system** (helps the body control and prevent infections).

- **Stimulates increased production of alpha-1 and alpha-2 gamma globulins** (these prevent viral and other infections).

- **Interferon-like action** (helps prevent and control viral infections).

- **Promotes general cellular immunity**

- **Stimulates killer t-cells**

- **Inhibits tumor growth**

- **Fights viruses**

- **Fights candida** (see following section).

each of these different compounds, called *constituents*, and then test what medicinal effect each has, if any. They also look to see if these constituents are unique to a particular plant or common in many plants, because if a constituent occurs only in one plant, then we can more readily prove that it is this constituent, and no other, which is at least partly responsible for a particular medicinal effect.

Now although some herbalists are not in the least interested in the study of chemical constituents—and indeed one can be a good practitioner without knowing all these scientific details— still, correlating constituents with specific physiological effects has certain benefits. For one thing it expands our general knowledge.

But more importantly, for pragmatic purposes, it helps us to make better herbal preparations. When we know what compounds should be present in an herb, we can determine whether a given sample is the correct herb, and whether it has been grown, processed, and prepared in the best possible way. For while there are many fine manufacturers of herbal products, the sad fact is that with herbs, as with anything else, there are always unscrupulous people who care more about profit than quality. Or, on the other hand, some manufacturers may have good intentions but faulty information about the most up-to-date practices for producing effective medicines or simply be using old, worn-out herbs to begin with. There is an old saying: "garbage in, garbage out."

A tremendous amount of work has been done on the constituents of echinacea. Chemists have isolated scores of compounds, some of them unique to different echinacea species. Often they have also succeeded in linking these compounds with specific physiological effects and activities. Although a full description of this chemistry would be too detailed for a general work such as this one,** for our purposes here we can say that these compounds are divided into two general classes: water-soluble and fat-soluble compounds. Table 3 shows the main

---

**For those interested in a complete review of the chemistry, pharmacology, pharmacy, and extensive history of use of echinacea (including ethnobotany), see my book on the subject, *The Echinacea Handbook* (See reference #2).

types of active compounds found in these two classes for the three major commercial species of echinacea.

Leading researchers feel that both the water-soluble polysaccharides and cichoric acid, as well as the fat-soluble compounds (like isobutylamides and polyacetylenes), boost the body's immune response.[12,13] Professor Wagner, one of the world's leading experts on medicinal plants, believes that the *polysaccharides* (large sugar molecules) are responsible for much of echinacea's immune-potentiating effect.[14] He also believes these compounds stimulate the fibroblasts, inhibit hyaluronidase, and induce interferon—effects which all enhance the body's ability to fight bacterial and viral infections. According to Wagner's theory, the mechanism for these actions would be due to the structure of echinacea's polysaccharides, which greatly resembles that of major compounds in the cell walls of many bacteria. Thus when the body senses the presence of polysaccharides, it may "mistake" them for bacteria and start to build up the immune system. This activity is like an exercise or drill for many immune functions of the body.

However, Rudolph Bauer, an associate of Wagner's, feels that the fat-soluble components of echinacea are more responsible for the plant's remarkable immune activity.[15] It is the isobutylamides of the fat-soluble constituents which give fresh and recently dried echinacea its sharp, tingling taste—that "zing" which some herbalists take as the sign of good echinacea. Although echinacea's polysaccharides do indeed show strong activity, Bauer points out that they may not necessarily be the most important active compounds for a couple of reasons. First of all, compounds very similar to echinacea's polysaccharides are found in a wide range of plants, especially in the daisy family. Second, polysaccharides may be broken down in the digestive tract before they can even be absorbed into the blood.

Of course, it is conceivable that immune stimulation may take place in the mouth, where immune tissue is activated immediately by contact with polysaccharides. However, this theory in turn is disputed, since the alcohol in tinctures may destroy the potency of echinacea's polysaccharides.

Table 3			
The Active Compounds of Echinacea			
Fraction	**E. purpurea**	**E. angustifolia**	**E.pallida**
Oil-soluble	Isobutylamides	Isobutylamides	Polyacetylenes
Water-soluble	Cichoric Acid Polysaccharides	Echinacoside Polysaccharides	Echinacoside Cynarin

As you can see, like so many other things in life, we do not yet know everything there is to know about echinacea's active ingredients—but we do know enough to create excellent and consistent echinacea products right now.

Echinacea preparations have a solid track record in clinical and laboratory studies, and thousands of doctors currently use them for a long list of infectious diseases.

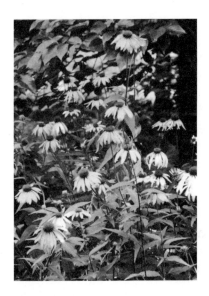

Fig. 3   Echinacea purpurea

A patch of wild plants growing in the garden.

WHAT CONDITIONS IS ECHINACEA BEST FOR?

This is, naturally, the practical question that most readers will want answered, and it is a good question. As it turns out, echinacea is ideal for what is called in Traditional Chinese Medicine "surface conditions," that is, illnesses that come and go and are not deeply seated or chronic. Colds and flu are classic examples of surface conditions, as are abscesses, bronchitis, sore throats, and many other common infections, if they are not chronic. For such conditions our immune systems have cells called *macrophages* (this means, literally, "big eaters") that quickly migrate to the site of infections to stop bacteria, viruses, and other pathogens from gaining a foothold, or to eliminate them once they have already entered into the body. Tests show that echinacea greatly stimulates these macrophages and increases their effectiveness. (see fig. 4, p.18)[16,17,18]

I have found that children respond especially well to echinacea.

Another very important use of echinacea is for candidiasis. Recent controlled studies demonstrated that a fresh liquid preparation of echinacea, taken orally, caused a marked reduction in recurrences of candidal colpitis and/or vulvitis (vaginal yeast infection).[19]

Table 4 lists the major conditions for which echinacea has been clinically tested and found to be effective. Herbalists, acupuncturists, chiropractors, naturopaths, medical doctors, and other health practitioners commonly use echinacea to treat these ailments. Be sure to review them carefully, since there was not room to list them all in the text. Also, be sure to review the accompanying Table 5, which explains the dosages suggested for treating each of the conditions in Table 4.

The only thing I can add is that the overwhelming consensus of my own experience plus the testimony of friends, patients, and acquaintances, is that proper and regular use of echinacea can be effective for most of these conditions, especially when combined with rest, a high-quality diet and other healthy habits. I have also found that children respond especially well to echinacea.

However, my research and experience indicate that echinacea may not be the herb of choice for long-term or profound immune deficiencies, such as cancer, AIDS, or chronic fatigue syndrome (Epstein-Barr virus). In both Traditional Chinese Medicine (TCM) and Ayurveda (a traditional system of medicine from India), it is known that surface conditions are treated with one class of herbal formulas and profoundly deficient states with another.[20] Herbs such as *Astragalus membranaceous, Ligustrum lucidum, Panax ginseng,* and many fungi (especially reishi, *Ganoderma lucidum*) are used in these latter cases.[21,22,23] I call them "bone-marrow reserve" or "deep defense" builders and correlate them with the TCM concept of "Wei Chi tonics" or "protective vitality" builders. Echinacea can be used in conjunction with these other herbs for deeper-acting tonic formulas. (see fig. 4, p.18)

A good example of the difference between the surface and deep immune system was highlighted in a German study with children who were undergoing radiation and chemotherapy for cancer. One side-effect of drug and radiation treatment is the severe reduction of the white blood cell count, which is unfortunate since it is precisely white blood cells which must fight the spread of cancer. In this study, the researchers were happy to find that an echinacea preparation helped restore the white blood cell count in most of the children. However, they also noted that a few of the children did *not* respond to the echinacea preparation because their immune systems were too depleted on a deep level. In other words, they had no more "bone marrow reserve" (all of our immunologically-active cells originate in the bone marrow). Happily the echinacea eventually worked once the children were allowed to rest for a long time to nourish their bone-marrow reserves.[24] There is mounting evidence that the bone-marrow reserve builders mentioned above can help the bone marrow to create more immune fighters.[25]

One of the most important uses for echinacea seems to be to forestall or shorten the common cold, flu, and related ailments.

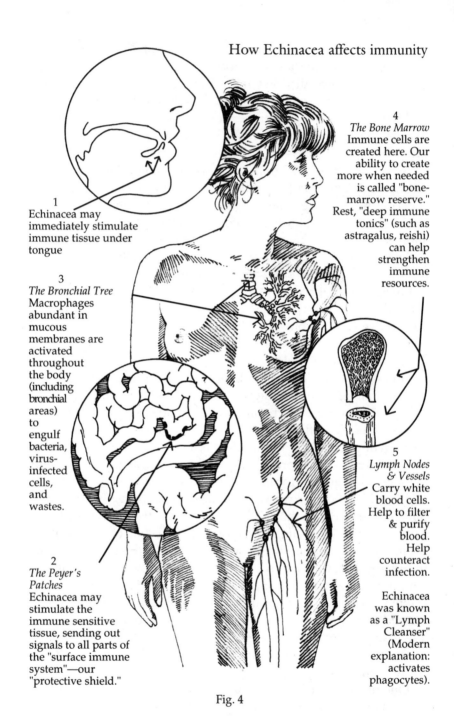

1
Echinacea may immediately stimulate immune tissue under tongue

3
The Bronchial Tree
Macrophages abundant in mucous membranes are activated throughout the body (including bronchial areas) to engulf bacteria, virus-infected cells, and wastes.

4
The Bone Marrow
Immune cells are created here. Our ability to create more when needed is called "bone-marrow reserve." Rest, "deep immune tonics" (such as astragalus, reishi) can help strengthen immune resources.

5
Lymph Nodes & Vessels
Carry white blood cells. Help to filter & purify blood. Help counteract infection.

Echinacea was known as a "Lymph Cleanser" (Modern explanation: activates phagocytes).

2
The Peyer's Patches
Echinacea may stimulate the immune sensitive tissue, sending out signals to all parts of the "surface immune system"—our "protective shield."

Fig. 4

Table 4

Main Uses of Echinacea

General infections and wound healing	use echinacea topically and internally (see table 5); internally add garlic
Colds or flu	especially before onset or in early stages, take a *protective* dose (see Table 5 for dosage guidelines). Take a *full course* when experiencing aggravated symptoms; if desired, put drops in ginger tea or sage and lemon peel tea
Candidiasis	for an acute situation, take a *full course*; for long-term use (up to several months), a *tonic dose;* add black walnut, garlic and pau d'arco
Strep throat	use *full course* as a gargle, then swallow solution combined with usnea liquid extract;[26] add propolis
Staph infections (impetigo, under nails,etc.)	take *protective dose* internally; apply locally full strength with usnea liquid extract
Urinary tract infections	for cystitis and urethritis especially, take a *full course*, as needed, followed by *maintenance dose* for 2 weeks; put drops in a tea of marshmallow root, licorice and pipsissewa; add usnea

---

Pelvic Inflammatory Disease (P.I.D.)	*full course* at *maximum dose,* stop for 3 days, then take another course as needed; *maintenance dose* for up to a month; rest and a nourishing diet are essential; do sitz baths daily
Tonsil and non-strep throat infections	use *protective dose* as a gargle, then swallow solution; use drops in sage tea; add usnea
Upper respiratory tract infections	put diluted solution of tea or tincture in nasal spray bottle and spray on back of throat several times a day; take *full course* internally; may use with grindelia and yerba santa herb or extract
Infected wounds	keep area moist with tincture, full strength; take internally; may use with comfrey poultice externally
Burns	*use maintenance dose* topically and internally; may be used with calendula cream
Herpes	use commercial creams or full-strength tincture topically; internally use a *protective dose* during acute phases, and a *tonic dose* thereafter, especially during times of stress

Skin ulcers

keep the area moist with tincture (full strength)

Psoriasis

take maintenance dose internally, and apply externally; add milk thistle extract internally

Whooping cough

full course during acute phases. For children under 5, reduce dose to 10 drops 3-5x/ day; for ages 6-10, 20 drops 3-5x/day: for 11-16, 1 dropperful 3-5 x/day; may add drops in thyme tea with a little goldenseal

Bronchitis

take *full course* internally; may add grindelia andyerba santa or add to elecampane ($^1/_2$), marshmallow (1) and licorice ($^1/_4$) parts

Leucopenia (low leucocyte count) and low t-helper cell levels

take *full course*; however, this treatment works only for leucopenia due to radiation therapy and other causes not directly related to long-term deficiency of immune function and general nutri- tion, malabsorption, or abusive life-style; astragalus, codonopsis, ligustrum and reishi tea or commercial product can be taken concurrently for up to 9 months for deeper immune strengthening

Rheumatoid arthritis	take *tonic dose* for anti-inflammatory effect; try taking a feverfew tablet everyday (see my article for more information)[27]
Allergies	take *tonic dose* for food allergies, environmental sensitivity, hay fever, and any other allergies not related to long-term immune deficiency; can be used with goldenseal and eyebright tea or extract
Toothaches and mouth and gum infections	gargle and swish extract, then swallow; apply full-strength to infected area 3-5 times daily; may add propolis or myrrh liquid extract
Bites and stings (insects, animals—rattlesnakes)	apply full strength on the bite and take internally
Blood and food poisoning	take large doses internally (1-4 droppersfull, or 4 capsules, every 2 hours)
Boils, carbuncles, abscesses	apply externally, and take *full course* internally
Eczema	use *maintenance dose* internally; may use with *Viola tricolor* liquid extract

HOW TO USE ECHINACEA

When taking Echinacea for the first time, always start with a low dose for a few days, to assure that there is no individual sensitivity. Then the dose can be gradually increased to full dose.

Table 5

Suggested Dose Schedule

Type of Dose	Quantity	Duration
Tonic Dose	10 drops/day of tincture 2 capsules/day 1 tablet/day	up to 9 months, as needed
Maintenance Dose	20 drops 2X/day of tincture 2 capsules 2X/day 1 tablet 2X/day	up to 2 months
Protective Dose	1 dropperful 2-3 X/day 2 capsules 3-4X/day 2 tablets 2X/day	10 days on, 4 days off, for up to 3 cycles
Full Course	1-2 droppersful every 2 hrs. 3-4 capsules every 2 hrs. 1-2 tablets every 2 hrs.	10 days maximum, then use protective dose
Children's Dose	under 6: 10 drops max/dose 7-10: 20 drops max/dose 11-13: 30 drops max/dose 14-16: 1 dropperful max/dose	same as above, depending on severity of the condition

There are good reasons to assume that echinacea works best during a ten-day course. German researchers have found that the stimulation of phagocytosis (one important parameter of immune activation) lasts only 10 days, both with oral doses and when injected.[28,29] After this time, the immune system may become accustomed to large doses—and at least the enhanced phagocytosis, an important aspect of blood purification, drops to just above normal. This corresponds with my own experience. Interestingly, the German researchers found that the maximum immune stimulation came between 3 to 6 days after the first dose was taken. In other words, echinacea may take at least one day before it "kicks in." That is why it is best to begin taking it immediately when one feels a cold or flu (or any other infection) "coming on."

I believe that this research suggests three things.

1) Take large doses of echinacea only when needed, not as a matter of course.
2) Take small 10-15 drop doses (per day) of echinacea for up to 9 months to "exercise" the surface immune function or "protective shield."
3) If large doses are required over a longer period than 10 days, try taking the echinacea in cycles—10 days on and 5 days off.

It has been my experience that it is important to keep taking echinacea for 48 hours after the symptoms of a cold, flu or infection disappear—or a relapse may occur.

For external application, use echinacea salve or ointment (available commercially); or apply the liquid extract to a cotton pad and fix it in place; or make a tea of the root or leaves and apply in a similar fashion. Be sure to change the dressing often for acute infections.

The above conditions are ones that the author has either seen echinacea work for first-hand, or in a few cases they are ones commonly treated with echinacea by eclectic or German doctors. However, no herbal remedy will work for everyone 100% of the time. Also, any natural remedy works better when combined with healthy habits.

IS ECHINACEA SAFE?

This is the next question that people usually ask, and the answer is overwhelmingly Yes. Tests performed on *E. purpurea* have demonstrated it to be completely non-toxic and nonmutagenic.[30] That is the beauty of this natural antibiotic. In my personal experience, I have found no side effects during seven years of regularly taking a 50% water and alcohol extract of fresh *E. angustifolia* roots. Once I took a full ounce of the preparation at one time. However, I have heard several reports of minor skin rashes resulting from use of the tincture,[31] and one report concerning throat irritation from drinking the tincture straight from the bottle. (This can be counteracted by diluting the tincture in water or other liquid before taking a dose, especially for children.)

WHAT IS THE BEST KIND OF ECHINACEA PREPARATION?

There are four major kinds of echinacea preparations that are commonly available.

1. Raw plant (whole, powdered, or "cut and sifted")
2. Liquid extracts, or tinctures
3. Powdered extracts
4. Products that contain echinacea in combination with other herbs (such as golden seal).

All of these can be of high quality, provided one knows how to choose them. The key questions one should keep in mind when selecting any echinacea products from the shelves of herb stores, natural foods stores, or other sources, are the following:

✔ What species of echinacea, or combination of species, does the product contain?
✔ What is the quality of the herbs contained in the product?
✔ How is the product prepared?

The Species of Echinacea

Although there are nine different species of echinacea that grow wild in this country (all east of the Rockies), only three have a history of use and clinical testing. Hence only these three are commonly sold in health food stores and herb shops: *Echinacea angustifolia* (narrow-leaved coneflower), *Echinacea purpurea* (purple coneflower), and *Echinacea pallida* (pale coneflower). Refer to Table 6 and figures 1A, 3 and 6 to help you distinguish between these species.

Naturally people often ask me which of these three main species is the best to use. After reviewing the world's literature and using several different species myself for many years, I feel that *E. angustifolia* and *E. purpurea* are equally beneficial.

Table 6

The Main Species of Echinacea[32]

Species	Appearance
Echinacea purpurea	tall and stout, with wide leaves; large purple flowers with a high (1-2") cone; yellow pollen; grows scattered in eastern states
Echinacea pallida	smaller, with narrow leaves; pale purple petals; white pollen; grows in northern plains states
Echinacea angustifolia	shortest plant, with narrow leaves; shorter petals, not so drooping; grows in middle to lower plains states

Echinacea angustifolia roots have a long history of use by John Uri Lloyd, the first echinacea product manufacturer in this country. He made a success of a high-alcohol, highly concentrated liquid extract called "Echafolta". This preparation had many years of effective use by doctors in the early 1900's.

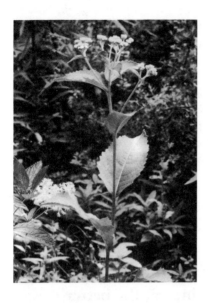

Fig. 5 *Parthenuim integrifoluim*

A common adulterant of Echinacea purpurea, known as "prairie dock."

But *E. purpurea* has a great track record, too. Dr. Gerhard Madaus began manufacturing a liquid from the tops of this plant, when seeds he received from America turned out to be the wrong kind. He was expecting *E. angustifolia*, and was thus disappointed, but later found that *E. purpurea* worked quite well in its own right.

As for *E. pallida*, it is often sold as *E. angustifolia*, both in this country and in Europe. According to Dr. Bauer, probably the world's leading authority on the chemistry of echinacea, *E. pallida* has immune-stimulating properties, but some of its important constituents may break down faster than in the other species, and its roots contain fewer of the important immune active amides.[33] Among herbalists there seems to be a consensus that *E. pallida* works, though it is not as desirable as the other two.

Steven Foster, author of *Echinacea Exalted*[34]—an informative book well worth getting for those interested in further study—has this to say about the matter:

> *E. pallida* is, "Traditionally not considered as good as the other 2 species of echinacea."

When I asked him what he thought about *E. angustifola* and *E. purpurea* having higher concentrations of the amides, he answered,

> "It's clear that the efficacy of *Echinacea* is not due to a single active component. Besides, much of what has been sold as *E. angustifolia* is in fact *E. pallida*, which is a highly variable plant. Until a great deal more clearly defined research is conducted, any conclusions on *E. pallida* are subjective generalities at best."

The conclusion seems to be, "keep an open mind," though Foster did say that *E. angustifolia* was his own personal favorite among the three species. When I asked him why, he answered, "I like the flavor."

Basically, the fresher the echinacea, the better it is.

Today, the best-studied preparations of echinacea are liquid concentrates of the tops of *E. purpurea*. Some say this is no coincidence, since E. purpurea is by far the easiest species to cultivate and gives the highest yields. Thus perhaps the other species make just as good medicine, but simply haven't been studied as much. Still, because *E. angustifolia* was the preferred species in this country for many years—first by the Eclectics and later by various herbalists—many modern manufacturers mix the roots of *E. angustifolia* with the tops of *E. purpurea*. This makes for a more complete blend. Some companies even add the seeds or flowers of either species, probably because the seeds give a biting, tingling taste to the preparation which has often been taken as a sign of high quality herb.

What this all means, in pragmatic terms, is that when buying echinacea products, you want to be sure that you are getting pure *E. angustifolia* **and** *E. purpurea*, not other species of echinacea or even completely different herbs. Recently I worked closely with an analytical laboratory in testing many of the commercially available echinacea products for purity, and we found that supposed *E. angustifolia* products often contained a mixture of *E. angustifolia* and *E. pallida*.[35] And the situation with *E. purpurea* was even worse—it was commonly adulterated with *Parthenium*, a plant that is not even a species of echinacea and has little medicinal value! Thus it is a good idea to buy only "Certified Organically Grown" echinacea, because it is almost guaranteed not to be adulterated.**

Wild vs. Cultivated Species

A subcategory of the discussion about which species of echinacea to use concerns the question of whether the wild or cultivated species are better. The widespread rumor that wild echinacea is stronger than its cultivated counterpart is precisely

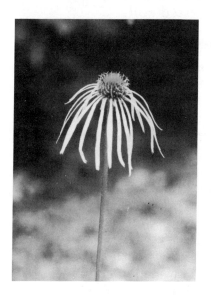

Fig. 6 *Echinacea pallida*

A common adulterant of "wildcrafted" *E. angustifolia*.

**The problem of adulteration is widespread, but not hopeless. The rise of small, family-owned enterprises dealing in certified organic or wildcrafted herbs during the last decade has helped create a quality-consciousness in the industry. Also, the American Herbal Products Association (AHPA) recently forged a tentative accord among members who are manufacturers and distributors to stop selling adulterated products.

that—nothing more than a rumor. There is not an ounce of clinical or laboratory evidence to support this claim. In fact, there is every reason to believe that carefully grown organic echinacea will be of a more consistent quality than wild echinacea that happens to grow in poor soil or is subjected to adverse weather conditions. Also, as our knowledge of the chemistry and pharmacology of echinacea grows, it is not inconceivable that someday we may, with breeding techniques, be able to create more potent strains of echinacea. These kinds of innovations over "the wild" have already had spectacular results with wheat, rice, corn, and other major food crops.

If you buy certified organic products.....the herb is grown in living rather than lifeless, sterile or devitalized soil.

The truth of the matter is that there are some very compelling reasons *not* to buy wild echinacea—one of the main ones being to preserve our wilderness. For the last 100 years (or so) wildcrafters have been digging between 50-100,000 pounds of echinacea annually for exportation to Europe—and this may be a conservative estimate. I have heard that there are still vast fields of wild echinacea in places, but, considering that the plant's native range land has mostly been destroyed, developed, or over-grazed, it seems likely that these wild populations will soon be endangered. For instance, one species of echinacea, *E. tennesseensis*, was considered extinct until a small population was discovered in an open cedar glade in Davidson County, Tennessee.[36] For this reason I strongly encourage organic, commercial cultivation not just of echinacea but of most medicinal plants and use only organically cultivated echinacea (both *E. purpurea* and *E. angustifolia*) in my own formulas.

Another good and practical reason to avoid wild echinacea is that the government does not regulate the wildcrafting industry very well; hence there is no legal guarantee of any kind for the label "wild." Many products are sold that claim to be "wild *E. purpurea*," which is impossible, because *E. purpurea* grows too sparsely to be collected from the wild. It is all commercially cultivated in the western United States and in Europe.

If you buy certified organic products, on the other hand, you can be sure that the herb is grown in living, rather than lifeless, sterile or devitalized soil, and that no pesticides or herbicides were used (these, ironically, may suppress the immune function). Products that contain organic echinacea are not much more expensive than products that do not contain it, and often they cost the same. Guidelines for using the name "organic" or "certified organic" vary from state to state, but a national law is imminent and may soon be a reality.

How to Determine Quality

Basically, the fresher the echinacea, the better it is. Some manufacturers go to great lengths to preserve freshness—they will even make liquid or powdered extracts of the plants right from the field. It has been known for a long time that echinacea roots lose their potency when exposed to air, warmth, or moisture for more than a few months (in some cases exposure even for weeks is enough to ruin the herb). This is especially true of the cut or powdered herb. Thus, if you buy bulk echinacea from an herb store, make sure to buy the whole root instead of the powdered

---

Dried whole root retains its active properties very well.

---

herb, or at least large pieces of the root. Powdered herb in capsules or tablets can also degrade (because both plastic bottles and gelatin capsules breathe), though obviously less quickly than bulk powder. Capsules packed in glass bottles last longer than those packed in plastic ones.

Table 7
Expected Shelf Life for Echinacea

Preparation	Shelf Life
Whole leaf	1/2 to 1 year
Whole root	1 to 2 years
Cut and sifted root	1 year
Powdered herb, capsules	1 to 1 1/2 years
Powdered herb, coated tablets	1 to 2 years
Powdered extract, capsules	1 1/2 to 2 years
Liquid extract (tincture)	2 to 3 years

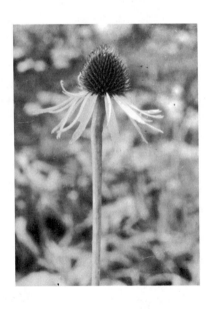

Fig. 7 *Echinacea parodoxa*

The only yellow-flowered Echinacea. Not sold commercially, unless as an adulterant of wildcrafted *E. angustifolia.*

Of course, there are always pros and cons. Two good reasons to buy capsules are that they are convenient and cost-effective. So if you do opt for capsules, look at the *manufacture* date (not the expiration date) stamped on the bottle. Try to buy bottles that are as recent as possible and never more than one year old. If a bottle has no date on it, it is better not to buy it since there is no way to know how old the herb is. If you can only find the

Echinacea

Table 8

The Pros and Cons of Echinacea Preparations

Preparation	Advantages	Disadvantages
Whole root or herb	holds freshness for over a year, if stored properly; cost effective	must be ground or powdered before use; less convenient
Cut and sifted	ready for making tea; cost effective	loses quality faster than whole root; less convenient than patent products
Capsules or tablets of powdered root	convenient; cost effective	best to use before 1 1/2 years; not as concentrated
Freeze-dried preparations	preserves freshness	can absorb moisture; shelf-life may be reduced[38,39]
Liquid extracts (tinctures)	hold quality for over 2 years; convenient; fairly cost effective; work fast	some people object to alcohol; glycerin can be irritating if not diluted
Powdered or concentrated extract	potent; convenient; no taste when in capsule or tablet	not so cost effective; not as quick-acting as liquids

expiration date, ask the store owner or call the manufacturer to find out how long the expiration date is from the date of manufacture, and do your math!

The most durable type of echinacea preparation is liquid extracts or *tinctures.* These retain their potency for up to two or even three years, especially when stored in amber bottles, away from heat and light. The main drawback of tinctures, however, is that their alcohol content may irritate or not be acceptable to some people. In this case the drops can be highly diluted in water or juice or placed in boiled water to evaporate much of the alcohol. Table 7 shows the normal shelf life, in my experience, for the major commercial preparations of echinacea (assuming favorable storage temperature, low light levels, and normal humidity), and Table 8 lists the general pros and cons of the major commercial preparations of echinacea.

How the Product is Prepared

This issue concerns the more technical aspects of the factors that contribute to quality discussed above; it is not as critical to the average consumer, though it may be of interest.

...we do not yet know everything there is to know about echinacea preparations. Even if there is a "golden recipe" to be discovered, it may well be many years before we find it.

Bauer found that dried whole root of echinacea retains its active properties very well—much better than powder.[37] However, because of the amount of cellulose and lignin present in the whole root, a concentrated extract may be more effective in the amounts generally recommended with commercial preparations (1-3 capsules or tablets, 2-3 X/day). Apparently the extraction process also releases constituents from cell walls, which may make extracted preparations more assimilable by the digestive tract. But, on the other hand, we do not yet know that sensitive constituents are not lost due to the heat of the extraction process itself. For this reason, most herbalists feel that the best preparations use as little heat as possible for the extraction process—pluses for cold-processed tinctures, freeze-dried and shade-dried preparations.

In simple language, all this just means that we do not yet know everything there is to know about echinacea preparations. Even if there is a "golden recipe" to be discovered, it may well be many years before we find it. In the meantime, when all is said and done, it is my experience that if the herb used is of good quality, and if it is processed soon after harvest, then the product will be effective. The details of what ratio of ethanol-to-water is best; whether dried, freeze-dried, or fresh herb is best; and whether *E. purpurea*, *E. angustifolia*, *E. pallida*, or some other untested species is best—all of these questions may well be fine-tuning.

Growing Echinacea

Find seeds or small plants of echinacea in a nursery and grow them yourself. *Echinacea purpurea* is the easiest to grow. It will do well in nearly any climate, but does not prefer hot, dry areas. If you live in such a climate, grow the plants in partial shade, or keep them well-watered. *E. angustifolia*, a native to the plains, prefers hot summers and very cold winters. I have found that *E. angustifolia* does not do as well as *E. purpurea* in a coastal climate. *E. pallida* is not as fussy as *E. angustifolia*, and it grows more quickly and vigorously.

The easiest way to grow echinacea is to buy the plant already in a pot, which can be set out in rich, well-drained soil and mulched with compost. The tops of *E. purpurea* can be harvested throughout the summer; try eating a leaf daily as a mild immune "tonic"—the flavor is provocative and you might even like it!

The roots of any of the three species can be dug in the fall around the first freeze, after the tops have died back. Wash them and dry them well in a warm, shaded place with good air circulation and store whole for future use. For detailed information on the fine details of growing echinacea, including commercial cultivation, see my book *The Echinacea Handbook*.

By growing this beautiful plant, we are helping to preserve our precious wild resources and getting to know the plant first-hand— herbs always seem to work best this way.

A FEW COMMENTS BY HERBALISTS
WHO USE ECHINACEA

Ed Smith (Herbalist, Manufacturer, Williams, OR):
"Because of its potentiating effects on the body's immune system, Echinacea favorably influences a broad array of medical maladies and can often bring about rapid and complete healing where all else seems to fail.

No remedy, herbal or otherwise, *always* works, but I can say that in all my years of dispensing medicinal herbs, I have never seen an herb work as effectively, consistently and safely as Echinacea. It is *the* herb to convert the most ardent herbal skeptic."

Cascade Anderson Geller (Clinical Herbalist, Portland, OR):
"It is important to warm up echinacea—add a warming, stimulating agent in formulas, especially when used for acute infections; ginger, cayenne, cinnamon or prickly ash—my favorite because it's a native American plant. With some people it can have no effect in acute cases after taking large amounts, but it works best in combination with other herbs. Add golden seal and warming herbs, especially with mucous membranes (colds & flu).

Student case studies in the naturopathic clinic show that a combination works better."

Brian Weissbuch (Clinical Herbalist, San Anselmo, CA):
"Echinacea's primary indication is lymphatic stasis with inflammation and immune-depression. As exposure to environmental pollution increases, this herb becomes increasingly valuable. Bear in mind that universal panaceas are mythical creatures—echinacea is not for everyone."

Amanda McQuade (Clinical Herbalist, Santa Rosa, CA):
"Echinacea is deserving of its old name, prairie doctor.
I couldn't imagine not having it as a core of my herbal practice.

So I am encouraging all my clients to grow it, as the wild sources are being overpicked, to address our society's burgeoning interest in immune health, for which echinacea is a blessing from the earth."

Michael Tierra (Clinical Herbalist, Author of Way of Herbs):
"As a native perennial of the Great Plains, it is the very symbol of North American herbalism beginning with its use by the Native Plains Indians and continuing with the great Eclectic herb movement of the late 19th and early 20th centuries.

Energetically, echinacea has a cool energy with a bitter, pungent, slightly sweet flavor. From a Chinese medical perspective, it goes to the lungs and stomach which rule the "wei chi" (immune system) and the liver which is the organ of detoxification. It therefore is classified and used in the Chinese herb category of clearing heat and detoxifying.

Echinacea's prime area of effect is for hypermetabolic conditions of "damp heat", especially when there is yellowish pus. Being a cool, detoxyifying herb it has less value for conditions and constitutions that arise out of deficiency and internal coldness, as in the case of whitish or clear discharges. Therefore, one may not expect echinacea to work alone either in conditions of yin deficiency (auto-inflammatory, wasting diseases), or in mild conditions arising from internal coldness or low metabolism.

All parts of the plant are effective but the root should be preferred in cases which tend towards deficiency, while the aerial parts are effective for conditions which tend more toward excess."

Brigitte Mars (Herbalist, Alfalfa's Market, Boulder, CO):
"Echinacea is truly one of nature's important gifts. I have seen this herb help thousands of people avoid the overuse of antibiotics. There have been few, if any, side-effects and many health benefits. This is a plant we need to grow more of. It seems like people come into the store for the first time just for this one product."

REFERENCES

1. Lyons, A.B. 1907. *Plant Names Scientific and Popular.* Detroit: Nelson, Baker & Co.
2. Hobbs, C. 1989. *The Echinacea Handbook.* Box 742, Capitola, CA: Botanica Press.
3. Gilmore, A. 1911. Uses of Plants by the Indians of the Missouri River Region. *Bur. Amer. Eth. Ann. Rep.* 33: 368.
4. Bauer, R. 1989. Personal communication.
5. Lloyd, J.U. 1917. *A Treatise on Echinacea.* Cincinnati: Lloyd Bros. Reprinted by Herb Pharm, Williams, OR.
6. Ellingwood, F. 1898. *American Materia Medica,* Therapeutics and Pharmacognosy. Chicago: Chicago Medical Press. Reprinted by Eclectic Medical Publications, Portland, 1983.
7. Bauer, R. and H. Wagner. 1988. "Echinacea—Der Sonnenhut—Stand der Forschung." *Zeit Phytother* 9: 151.
8. Kleinschmidt, H. 1965. Study on reduction of infection in infants with Esberitox. *Ther. d Gegen.* 1258.
9. Helbig, G. 1961. Non-specific immune-therapy in infection prophylaxis. *Med. Klin.* 56: 1512.
10. Freyer, H.U. 1974. Frequency of common infection in childhood and likelihood of prophylaxis. *Forschrift der Ther.* 92: 165.
11. Amman, M. & K. Suter. 1987. Echinacea combination: effectiveness and compatibility in cases of flu and inflammation of the nose and pharynx. *Deut. Apoth.-Zeit.* 127: 853.
12. Bauer, R., et al. 1988a. Immunological *in vivo* and *in vitro* examinations of Echinacea extracts. *Arzn.-Forsch.* 38: 276.
13. Bauer, R. 1989. Influence of Echinacea extracts on phagocytotic activity. *Zeit. Phytother.* 10: 43.
14. Lohmann-Matthes, M. L. & H. Wagner. 1989. Macrophage activation by plant polysaccharides. *Zeit. Phytother.* 10: 52.
15. Bauer, R. 1989, op cit.
16. Lasch, H.G. 1983. The effect of Echinacin on phagocytosis and natural killer cells. *Die Med. Welt.* 34: 1463.
17. Wagner, H. & A. Proksch. 1985. *Economic and Medicinal Plant Research,* vol. 1. Orlando: Academic Press, p. 113.

18. Enbergs, H. & A. Woestmann. 1986. The effect of Echinacea angustifolia on phagocytic activity of peripheral leukocytes of rabbits. *Tierärztliche Umschau* 11: 878.
19. Coeugniet, E. & R. Kühnast. 1986. Recurrent candidiasis: adjuvant immunotherapy with different formulations of echinacin." *Therapiewoche* 36: 3352.
20. Bensky, D. & A. Gamble. 1986. *Chinese Herbal Medicine, Materia Medica.* Seattle: Eastland Press.
21. Bullock, C. 1984. Two Chinese herbs show blooming anticancer potential. *Texas Med. Trib.*
22. Wenbin, C., et al. 1983. *J. Trad. Chin. Med.* 3: 63.
23. James, J. 1986. AIDS *Treatment News* 19.
24. Chone, B. & G. Manidakis. 1969. Echinacin-test on leukocyte production in radiation therapy. *Deut. Med. Woch.* 27: 1406.
25. Guan, H.C. & Z. Cong. 1982. *Yaoxue Tongbao* 17: 177.
26. Hobbs, C. R. 1985. *Usnea and other medicinal lichens: the herbal antibiotics.* Box 742, Capitola, CA: Botanica Press.
27. Hobbs, C. 1989. Feverfew. *HerbalGram* 20: 26-36. (to order subscription or back issues: 1-800-373-7105)
28. Wagner, et al. 1988. Immunologische In-vitro-und In-vivo-Untersuchungen von Arzneiprä paraten. Phytotherapie. Stuttgart: Hippokrates Verlag, pp. 127-135.
29. Jurcic, K., et al. 1989. Two test-subject studies for the stimulation of granulocyte phagocytosis by Echinacea-containing preparations. *Zeit. Phytother.* 10 (2): 67-70.
30. Hobbs, *The Echinacea Handbook, op cit.*
31. Geller, C.A. 1988. Personal Communication.
32. McGregor, R.L. 1968. The Taxonomy of the Genus Echinacea (Compositae). *Univ. of Kansas Sci. Bul.* 48: 132.
33. Bauer, R. & P. Remiger. 1989. TLC and HPLC analysis of alkamides in *Echinacea* drugs. *Planta Med.* 55: 367-78.
34. Foster, S. 1986. *Echinacea Exalted,* 2nd rev. ed. Brixey, MO: Ozark Beneficial Plant Project.
35. Moring, S. & C. Hobbs. 1988. Unpublished results.
36. McGregor, *op cit.*
37. Bauer, R. 1987. Personal communication.
38. King, C.J. 1971. *Freeze-drying of foods.* Cleveland, OH: CRC Press.
39. Goldblift, F.A., ed. *Freeze-drying and advanced food technology.* New York: Academic Press.

Author's Disclaimer.

The information given in this book is for educational purposes and is not meant as a prescription for any ailment. If you have a serious illness, the author recommends seeking the services of a competent natural health practitioner. Unless a statement is specifically referenced, it could be the author's opinion, based on extensive study and personal experience.

NOTES

NOTES